Pain Reli

The Top 20 Psychoactive He. ai Remedies & Essential Oils For Instant Pain Relief

Table of content

Introduction

Pain is a fact of life for many people. It is something that everyone will experience at some point in their life. It can range from a simple headache to the pain of a broken bone or even nerve damage which can cause extensive long term issues. These types of pain can be triggered by one specific incident or can simply be a failure of your body's natural processes. The most basic understanding of pain suggests that it is a response to an issue; effectively you injure yourself and your body tells you that part of it is hurt. You can then take steps to deal with the issue.

However, whilst pain can be the result of a knock or a blow there are other occasions when you can experience phantom pain; this is the pain in a limb which you no longer have! Equally it is possible to place your body under extreme trauma and not feel any pain at all. These issues have helped scientists to clarify the reasons humans feel pain.

Many scientists now believe that pain is actually your body's way of telling you there is something wrong. Whilst this can be as obvious as a pain resonating from a specific injury, it can also be the result of internal damage which needs time to heal. In effect, the pain you feel can be seen as a warning symbol; it tells your body and your brain to protect a certain part of your body. One of the best examples of this is when you injure your back. The sharp pain you feel is the injury. However, the dull ache is your body protecting the injured area. It forces you to move differently and use alternative muscles. This allows the affected area to heal properly without being stressed.

Another benefit of pain is that it is the trigger for your body to produce a chemical known as opioids. These are actually the body's natural pain killers and will help to reduce the overall sensation of pain. There is also a school of thought that suggests that a pain receptor can switch into a constantly on mode after an incident of pain. The result of this is an increased sensitivity in the pain receptors which can result in long term pain; long after the injury should have healed itself.

There is no doubt that pain serves a valuable purpose. However, once you are aware of an issue it is generally beneficial for the pain to subside so that you may get on with the activities you need to do. This is why many people take painkillers. However, there can be an issue with painkillers; take too many and you may become reliant on them. As an alternative many people are turning to natural medicines; such as herbal treatment options or even essential oils.

These types of treatments have been used for hundreds and even thousands of years. Many Middle Eastern countries have a long history of alternate medicines and some of these can be as effective as any modern drug.

Chapter 1 – 10 Psychoactive Herbal Painkillers

There are actually a surprising number of psychoactive plants. These are any plant which can have a mind altering effect on your brain. However before you pick your favorite one and start feeling its benefits it is important to realize that are large number of these plants have addictive properties. You do not want to deal with your pain problems only to find you have an addiction problem!

1. *The Blue Lotus*

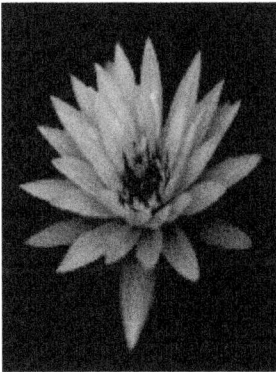

http://ep.yimg.com/ay/scents-of-earth/blue-lotus-oil-absolute-per-ml-sri-lanka-nymphaea-caerulea-17.png

The Blue Lotus is a stunning pale blue flower which is commonly known as an aphrodisiac. However, it can also be used as an effective pain killer. It is generally perceived to be one of the weaker types of painkiller but this can also be seen as a plus point in that it is less likely to create an addiction.

In fact, the mild psychoactive effects produced by this plant have often been linked with those trying to find a more divine state of mind. The Blue Lotus generally provides you with a warm feeling of contentment and you may feel slightly stimulated. However, alongside this it will provide relief from muscle spasm, cramps, severe headaches including migraines and, it has even been linked with reducing the effects of tinnitus

The best and possibly easiest way to consume this natural painkiller is by adding several flowers to a pot of boiling water. You can adjust the number of flours according to your personal tastes. You should bowl the flowers for approximately five minutes; you can then drink it hot or cold.

It is worth noting that the effects of this flower do not seem to improve or worsen if you consume large amounts of the flower.

2. *Kava Kava*

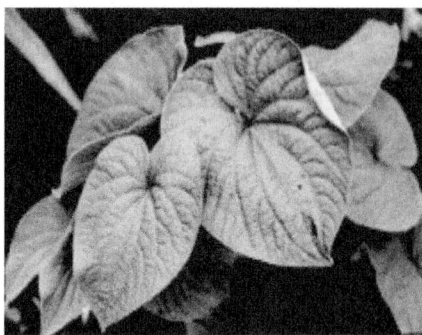

This herb was originally used by the Polynesians for a variety of purposes including pain relief. However, it has now become used commonly around the world. It has a light psychoactive effect on the body; mainly translating as a mood heightener. You are likely to feel anything is possible and the sky is the limit!

This herb is an effective pain reliever and has also been used as an effective local anesthetic; although this has now been replaced by medical professionals with modern drugs. Kava Kava has been shown to provide relief for anyone suffering from back pain; it is surprisingly effective. Alongside this it is a natural option to help with teething babies and can be used to help you sleep and reduce your levels of anxiety and stress.

Alongside offering pain relief it has been found to be effective at relieving the symptoms of bronchitis and can even counteract the effects of insect bites.

It is possible to purchase Kava Kava as a powder and dissolve two tablespoons in some water or even juice. It is possible to grind your own Kava Kava from the root of the plant. You will need to grind the root and mix it with some water before straining it through a fine mesh. The tighter the mesh the harder you will need to squeeze the kava through and the better the quality will be.

3. Lettuce

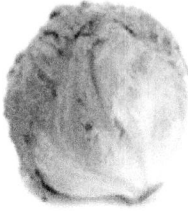

Lettuce that you can purchase in the local supermarket will not have a psychoactive effect on you or work as a painkiller. However, modern lettuce is a descendent of wild opium lettuce. This can still be found and even grown at home and is a much more powerful herb. As the name suggests, it is a relative of opium which you will probably have heard of. However, the opium lettuce is a milder form and was used extensively in the 1800's as a painkiller and even as a sedative.

It is also worth noting that although this is a relative of opium it has been shown to have the positive effects without side effects. The best way of consuming this is to use the sap from a fresh lettuce. You will need roughly one and a half grams of the sap in a cup of boiling water. It should be left to infuse for at least five minutes before you drink it. Sipping it allows the maximum effects of this pain killing psychoactive herb as it is absorbed into your bloodstream quicker.

Of course, being associated with the opium plant there are a range of psychoactive effects. In particular this will make you feel a little high and certainly happy.

4. Kratom

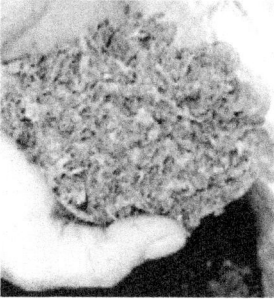

This herb actually comes from a tree in Southeast Asia; although it is now possible to grow it in a variety of other places. It has been used for many years by people in Asia as a stimulant and a sedative! Its effects depend upon the size of the dose. It has also been shown to be an effective painkiller and can be used to treat diarrhea.

There are two main methods of taking this herbal remedy. The first is by simply chewing the leaves fresh. It is advisable to wash them and remove the stringy middle vein first. The alternative is to dry the leaves and then crumble them. They should crumble easily once fully dried. Using this method will allow you to store the dried leaves in an airtight container for when you want them. To use them you simply place a teaspoon or two of the dried leaves in a cup of boiling water and leave it to brew for five minutes. This herb will make you feel good!

5. Marijuana

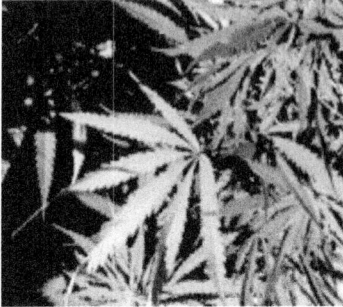

This is one of the more controversial and powerful painkillers that nature provides. Marijuana is well known for its mood altering effects. In general it acts as a muscle relaxant and stress reducer. In general people who take this natural herbal remedy will find themselves more relaxed and less inclined to react explosively to any situation. It is best described as being in a very 'chilled out' state. However, it is also important to check your local laws. Marijuana is not legal everywhere; although there are an increasing number of places recognizing the medical possibilities of this herb.

One of the biggest benefits is that it has been shown to be effective at reducing or eliminating pain even when traditional pain killers have no effect. The reason for this is simple; it works in a different way to prescription drugs. Marijuana causes the body to produce inhibitors which effectively block severe pain signals from being sent to the brain.

This is not a substance you should be growing at home; even if it is for personal pain relief. As it is illegal in many places you should only be able to get it through approved medical channels. The fact that it is still classified as a class one drug means that the research into this herb is limited.

6. Cannabis

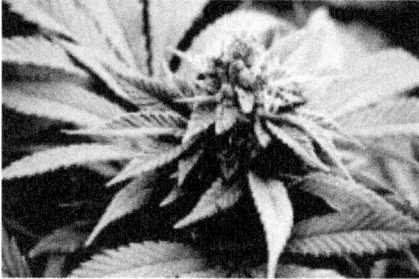

http://www.wakingtimes.com/wp-content/uploads/2015/01/Cannabis-Flower-1.jpg

This herb has been grown in various parts of the world for many years. There are records from the 18th and 19th centuries where patients have been prescribed cannabis to help relieve the pain of stomach cramps, treat anorexia and as a general painkiller.

For many years this herb was ignored as it is classified as an addictive substance and was not legal. Now, there is an increased interest in the potential of this as a medical aid. It has been shown to be exceptional beneficial to those with muscle spasms and has been seen to offer valuable relief; particularly to people suffering from multiple sclerosis.

The medically approved version has taken the leaves of the plant, dried them and crushed them before adding them to their medicine. There are people who simply smoke the herb to enjoy the mind altering effects. These are likely to include an elevated heart rate and a willingness to believe they can do anything.

Unfortunately it is difficult to predict the exact reaction. You will be likely to experience an ability to see brighter colors; mood changes; an inability to move your body correctly and you will struggle to think properly or solve any issues. It can even lead to hallucinations and paranoia; this is why it must be administered and monitored only by a medical professional.

Again, due to the sensitive legal nature of this herb it is not advisable to start growing it at home.

7. Phellodendron

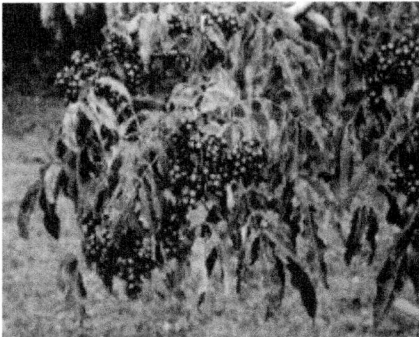

This beneficial herb is also known as Huang bai and is well established within the Chinese community. Interesting to be used effectively as a medicine you will need to locate one of the two species in the world. Generally they appear in North China and central China.

You can use the root of this plant, the berry, twigs or even the bark. Each of these parts needs to be ground into a fine powder which can then be encompassed in a pill or taken in powder form diluted in liquid.

Phellodendron has been shown to reduce stress and help settle your body. It has a sedative effect on you and your approach to life; this can reduce the pain in your body and even help you to sleep better. It is even used as an effective way of getting to sleep or having a good night's sleep and encourages muscle growth and repair as you rest. This is alongside the fact that it is an effective pain killer.

8. Chinese Cat Claw

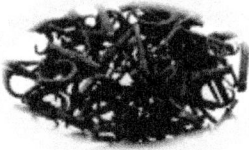

http://meridianbotanicals.com/images/Uncaria-Ramulus-Gou-Teng-sm.jpg

This herb has been around for many years but it has not been well known or use until very recently. It is also known as Gou Teng. In fact, research suggests that this amazing herb has been reducing the effects of the shakes accompanying Parkinson's disease, for thousands of years. It has also been shown to be an effective assistant in the fight against irritable bowel syndrome.

It comes from the stems and even the thorns of the Uncaria rhyunchophylla; it is best to harvest these parts during the autumn. The stems, with the thorns attached can be cut into small pieces and left to dry in the sunshine. You will then be able to crush or crumble the dried twigs and use them; either diluted in liquid or even mixed with food. It is recommended to only take a maximum of 30 grams each day as it will also have mind altering effects.

The herb has been shown to have an ability to reduce pain levels in the body. It is considered to be a relaxant, assisting your body to deal with a range of conditions. These include headaches, epilepsy (particularly in children), convulsions, fevers and even stomach disorders.

9. Red Sage Root

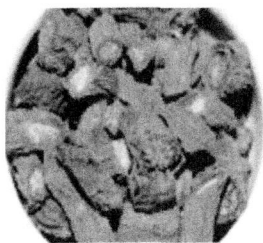

http://www.herbsandarts.com/site/cartpics/large/5918/red_sage_root_-_rs.jpg

This Chinese traditional medicine looks a lot like bark; it is often referred to as Chinese salvia and is, unsurprisingly, originally found in China. It is a perennial herb with red roots and large purple flowers. It is the root which provides the painkilling substance although it also has a range of other positive side effects.

It is worth noting that this herb should not be used if you have any issues with excess bleeding or suffer from regular nose bleeds.

To take this painkiller and general health booster you will need the root of the plant which must be dried and then crushed into a fine powder. This can then be used as a dry powder to make tea in the usual way. Drinking it in the form of tea is the fastest and most effective way of getting it into your body.

As well as providing pain killing effects this herb has been shown to be effective at improving circulation and even reducing fat within your arteries. It has even been suggested that it can reduce the possibility of gaining angina and actually regulate your heart better. It is known to be a relaxant and is likely to leave you feeling good as your aches and pains disappear.

10.California Poppy

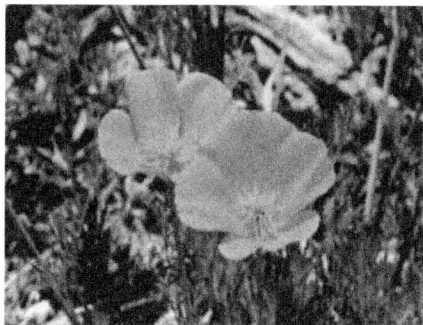

Unsurprisingly this herb is actually a poppy and is native to California. It has also been used for many years as a medicinal aid.

By itself it has been found to assist you with sleeping issues. This is because, as a psychoactive substance, it will help your mind enter a more relaxed, meditative state. In fact, it works in a similar way to Marijuana. Using this is likely to induce a relaxed state and ultimately you could even fall asleep! The actual outcome will depend upon you tolerance to the herb and your natural metabolism.

This is what has made is so good for insomniacs. However, it has also be found to benefit by relieving aches, anxiety and even with bladder or liver disease. There have even been reports of it benefiting those who frequently wet their bed.

Alongside this California Poppy can be mixed with a variety of other herbs to create an effective relief from nerve pain. It has also been used to reduce the effects of depression and even boost energy levels. In some ways the humble poppy could be the most powerful herb of all!

Chapter 2 – 10 Essential Oils to relive your Aches & Pains

Just as herbs have been used for thousands of years so have essential oils. These oils have proved to be extremely effective at dealing with a wide array of different types of pain. Although modern prescription drugs are effective they can often lead to side effects and the human body usually becomes immune to their effects over time. If you include the potential side effects of prescription drugs it is easy to say that natural alternatives are generally safer and more effective.

When using essential oils you will find that only a small amount is necessary as they are potent remedies. The following essential oils can be used to provide effective relief from a wide variety of painful conditions; you may be surprised at just how effective they are:

1. Lavender

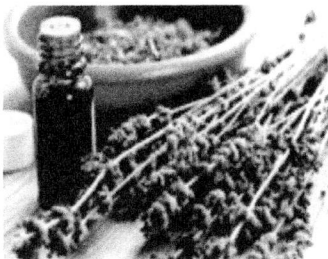

http://www.naturallivingideas.com/wp-content/uploads/2014/06/lavender-essential-oil.jpg

You will almost certainly have heard of lavender before and be familiar with the scent. However, you may not know that it can be very effective at relieving headaches; particularly those caused by tension, anxiety and migraines. Lavender essential oil is a mild sedative. It helps to soothe and calm the mind which will almost instantly make you feel calmer. This will assist in lowering your stress levels and reducing anxiety.

It is usually best to simply add a few drops of the oil to a bowl of hot water. You will then be able to hold your head over the bowl and breathe in the fumes. However, it is possible to put a drop of oil on your neck and one on your forehead. As ender essential oil is a fairly mild type of oil it is possible to do this without diluting it.

Lavender also acts as an anti-inflammatory. This means it can assist in removing any aches in your body; particularly if they are a result of muscle aches. To use it in this manner it is best to put three drops of oil with a tablespoon of coconut oil and then massage it into your skin at the source of the pain. It should start working within a few minutes.

2. Peppermint

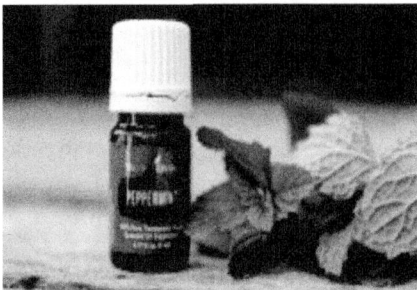

http://www.livingthenourishedlife.com/wp-content/uploads/2014/05/peppermint.jpg

Mints and specifically peppermint have been used for many years to provide pain relief. In fact, peppermint is used to supplement many types of cuisine as well as the aches and pains in your body. Peppermint essential oil is actually a combination of watermint and spearmint. You are certain to be familiar with this powerful scent.

Peppermint has traditionally been used to help with cases of indigestion. It is an effective relieving of trapped wind, bloat and nausea. The oil can also help to prevent your digestive system from spasms. In effect it has the ability to relax any and every part of your body. This helps to deal with muscle pains, nerve injury and even head pains. It is generally found within a range of medical products and can be taken safely this way. However, it is possible to put a couple of drops with a tablespoon of coconut oil to create excellent massage oil. This can give almost instant topically release when massaged gently into your skin.

Of course, peppermint is also very useful when you have a cold or blocked nose. You can sniff the oil or purchase one of the many peppermint products available; it is an exceptionally efficient decongestant.

3. Eucalyptus

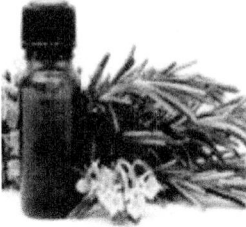

This oil has a well defined and distinctive aroma. It works in a similar way to peppermint and may even be a more effective decongestant. If you massage a couple of drops mixed with coconut oil into your skin you will notice an almost instant warming and soothing effect. The oil is too strong to apply to your skin undiluted as it is likely to burn. The only exception to this is if you have been bitten by an insect; one drop of the Eucalyptus essential oil will quickly remove the pain of the bite. Because the oil also has anti-inflammatory capabilities it will also help to ensure the bite does not swell or become infected. This is particularly beneficial if you have been bitten near an airway.

The oil is removed from the bark of the Eucalyptus tree and can also be found in its leaves. It is not one you would normally try to cultivate yourself. However, it is useful to keep some at home. When breathed in or applied to your nose it can help to clear your sinuses and relieve the dull ache that accompanies this congestion.

Eucalyptus essential oil is warming and will help to relax your muscles; this will reduce pressure on almost any injury and help to relieve the pain. It is surprisingly versatile oil.

4. Chamomile

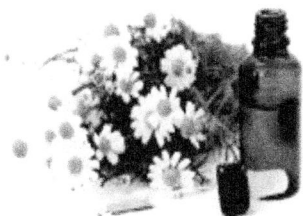

There are actually two main types of chamomile essential oil. One is German in origin and originates from the Matricaria chamomilla whilst the other is referred to as Roman and is located in the Anthemis noblis.

The Roman version is recognized as being milder. This means it is the better option if you need to treat children; especially if your child has an abdominal issue. Roman chamomile can be extremely effective at relieving the issue without irritating your child's sensitive digestive tract. The German version of this essential oil has been shown to have an impressive range of pain relieving functions; especially when dealing with inflamed areas. German chamomile has been found to very good at relieving lower back pain, PMS and even assisting in the treatment of bowel disease.

Both types of chamomile are effective at relieving muscles and joint pains. They are also good at reducing or even eliminating the pain that accompanies a bad headache.

Chamomile is also said to be relaxing for both your mind and body. This is why many people drink it regularly as a tea. Whilst this can help with overall health to benefit when treating the issues described above it is best to mix a few drops of chamomile oil with coconut oil and massage into the affected area.

5. Juniper

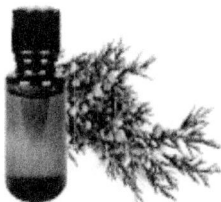

http://goodlivingessentialoils.com/wp-content/uploads/2014/10/juniper-berry-oil.jpg

The Juniper berry is a pale blue color. It is packed with essential oils which have proven to be very useful and effective at treating an array of conditions.

Juniper has been used with excellent results in the treatment of hemorrhoids and dysmenorrheal. It is a powerful oil which can quickly eliminate the pain associated with these conditions as well as digestion problems.

To relieve hemorrhoids it is advisable to put five or six drops of this oil into a hot bath and then relax for twenty minutes in the tub. The oil will gradually soak into your skin and the pain will gradually ease or even disappear.

You can also add a couple of drops to your favorite herbal tea or mix it with some olive oil. This can be consumed and will provide fast, effective relief from most digestive issues; including a buildup of gas.

Juniper is also a calming essential oil. You will notice that using it regularly will assist you in remaining calm in everyday events.

6. Ginger

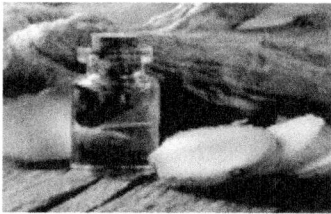

Ginger is an exceptionally popular substance. It is mixed with alcoholic drinks to add flavor and even drunk by itself on occasion. It can also be used in a variety of different recipes to improve the taste of a wide variety of delicacies.

However, it is also possible to extract some essential oil from a fresh ginger. This oil has become established as an excellent way to help reduce stomach issues. Ginger is commonly found in travel sickness products and in medications to smooth your digestive process. It is a powerful oil and research suggests you should consume no more than four grams of it per day.

Just like many of the other oils listed her you can massage this into your skin to create a topical relief from pain. However, it is generally better to mix two or three drops of this oil with a spoon of caster sugar as opposed to coconut oil. Wherever you apply it you will feel your skin warming and your muscles starting to relax. As well as being applied to your skin, it is completely safe to consume ginger.

This essential oil has been found to relieve the pain associated with illnesses such as arthritis, lupus and even multiple sclerosis. Whilst long term use of some essential oils can produce side effects this has not been found to be an issue with ginger.

7. *Sandalwood*

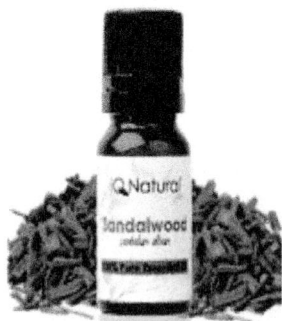

http://www.healthbenefitstimes.com/9/uploads/2014/12/Health-Benefits-of-Sandalwood-Essential-Oil.png

It is likely you will know the scent of sandalwood; it is one of the most popular for incense sticks which are frequently burnt around the house. The actual oil is located in the sandalwood tree but trees must be at least fifty years old to ensure they have quality oil.

This is actually one of the best pain relievers for almost any condition. It can be used effectively against muscle pain, skeletal pain and even the effects of neuralgia. The best way to administer this powerful oil is by adding three or four drops to a cup of boiling water. You can then allow the aroma to go into your sinuses and provide pain relief across your body. Alternatively you can drink this oil infused water; one cup every day will reduce pain and help you to feel one hundred percent again.

8. Clove

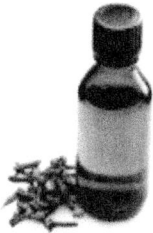

Cloves are frequently used in cooking but to add flavor. If you have ever bitten into one you will know they produce a burning sensation which quickly turns into a numb feeling. This makes them excellent at providing quick release from pain or even to be used as a local anesthetic.

The essential oil can be extracted from the cloves and stored for use as and when you need it. For instance, a drop of clove oil can be placed directly onto a source of toothache to provide instant relief. Alternatively you can put a few drops into a cup of water and gargle with it to help remove the pain of a sore throat.

In addition to this you can use clove oil in conjunction with other essential oils. For instance, clove oil mixed with jojoba oil can be massaged into any painful area on your body. This will warm the area and relax the muscles allowing pain relief from muscle pain and even joint pain.

Equally it can be used to deal with headaches; either when mixed with the jojoba oil or simply diluted with a little water.

9. Sweet Majoram

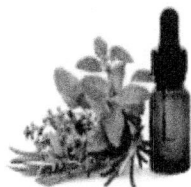

This essential oil has been found to have sedative properties. It is also an effective anti-inflammatory with an array of potential applications.

Research has shown that by mixing four drops of sweet majoram oil with the same amount of black pepper oil, lavender oil and peppermint oil you can make an oil which will provide very effective pain relief to any area of pain in the body. It has been used successfully by people with long term pain issues; they have reported dramatic reductions in pain after just a few weeks of regular use.

Just like clove oil, this essential oil can also be applied directly to a toothache and will provide instant release. It can be diluted with a little olive oil or coconut oil if you find it too strong by itself.

The mixture described above, or a simply mixture of sweet majoram and olive oil can be applied to your head and neck to relieve head pain, neck pain and even indigestion.

10.Bergamot

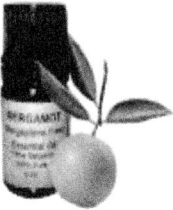

You may have already come across this essential oil; it is commonly used in Earl Gray tea to improve the flavor and help calm the mind. In fact, studies have shown that this oil is not only calming and reduces anxiety; it is also very effective at reducing the sensitivity of your nerves to pain. The easiest way to benefit from this stress reducing oil is simply to breathe the oil in; ideally put a few drops into a bowl of hot water and inhale the vapors. You will find that pain across your body reduces quickly.

It is a powerful oil and it is not advisable to apply it directly to your skin. However a few drops mixed with a teaspoon of olive oil or coconut oil can be used on your skin and will provide fast pain relief. It is particularly good with headaches and any stress related pain you encounter. Of course, this mixture can be applied anywhere on your body to provide effective pain relief.

Conclusion

For many years people have relied on the doctor and prescription medication to deal with pain issues; particularly chronic long term pain. However, this is not the only way of dealing with pain. There are many substances in nature which can be used to relieve symptoms of pain. Herbs and essential oils are the most obvious substances and have been used for thousands of years. In many cases these can have better long term effects as they have fewer side effects and the essential oils are non-addictive. Most of the herbs have the potential to be addictive but, with careful management, any addiction can be avoided.

It is important to note that essential oils are potent; care must be taken when handling them as undiluted oil can burn your skin. In addition, because they have powerful effects it is advisable to consult your doctor before you start using them; particularly if you are already on medication.

Essential oils are exceptionally good at relieving pain. However, the herbs often have the added benefit of being psychoactive. This means that they can alter your state of mind and help you to feel more relaxed whilst dealing with your pain. Most herbs and oils do not have any discernable side effects and it is perfectly possible to mix these two natural painkillers. However, as with anything you have not experienced before it is advisable to try them in a small dose first to ensure they are effective and safe for you to use.

Pain is something that many people live with for the long term as they are unable to find an effective pain reliever. This does not need to be the case. Although your body will build up a tolerance to prescription drugs which renders them useless; this does not happen with herbs and oils. These natural substances are simply accepted by your body and processed in the same way as any other food source.

There are a huge number of choices regarding oils and herbs which can offer you the pain relief you require. It is possible that you will need to experiment with what works best for your individual situation. Whilst most of the products listed in this book can provide excellent, almost instant relief for short term pain issues; longer term ones can require more specific mixtures. Every person is different and if you are dealing with long term pain it is advisable to try one combination for several weeks before moving onto a different one.

All the herbs and oils should be handled carefully; they are powerful substances and should never be left where children can access them. With proper precautions you can achieve the pain relief you have been craving!

FREE Bonus Reminder

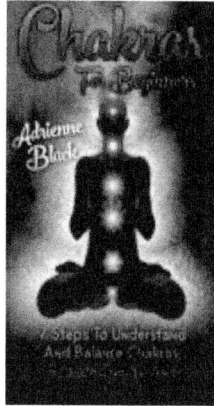

If you have not grabbed it yet, please go ahead and download your special bonus E book *"Chakras for Beginners. 7 Steps To Understand And Balance Chakras, Radiate Energy, And Strengthen Aura"*.

Simply Click the Button Below

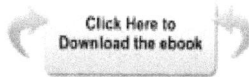

OR Go to This Page

http://lifehacksworld.com/free

BONUS #2: More Free & Discounted Books & Products

Do you want to receive more Free/Discounted Books or Products?

We have a mailing list where we send out our new Books or Products when they go free or with a discount on Amazon. Click on the link below to sign up for Free & Discount Book & Product Promotions.

=> **Sign Up for Free & Discount Book & Product Promotions** <=

OR Go to this URL

http://zbit.ly/1WBb1Ek

Printed in Great Britain
by Amazon